AF074972

This Book Belongs To

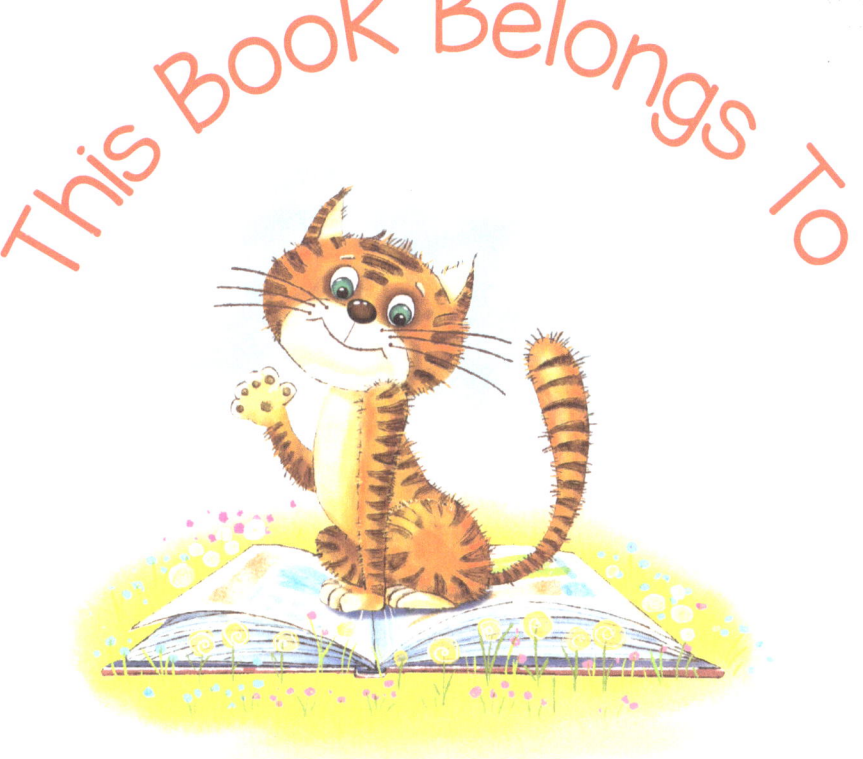

_____

_____

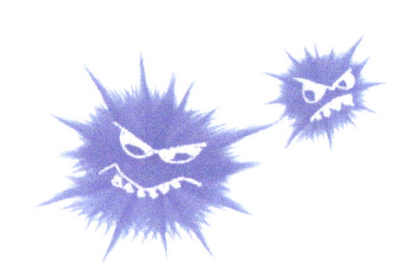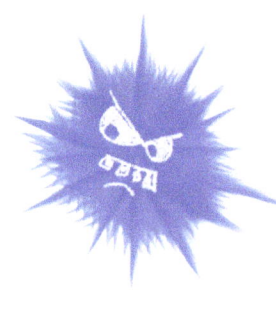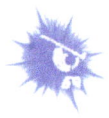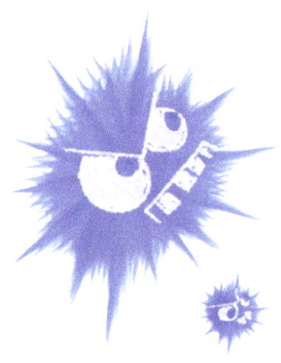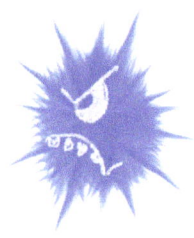

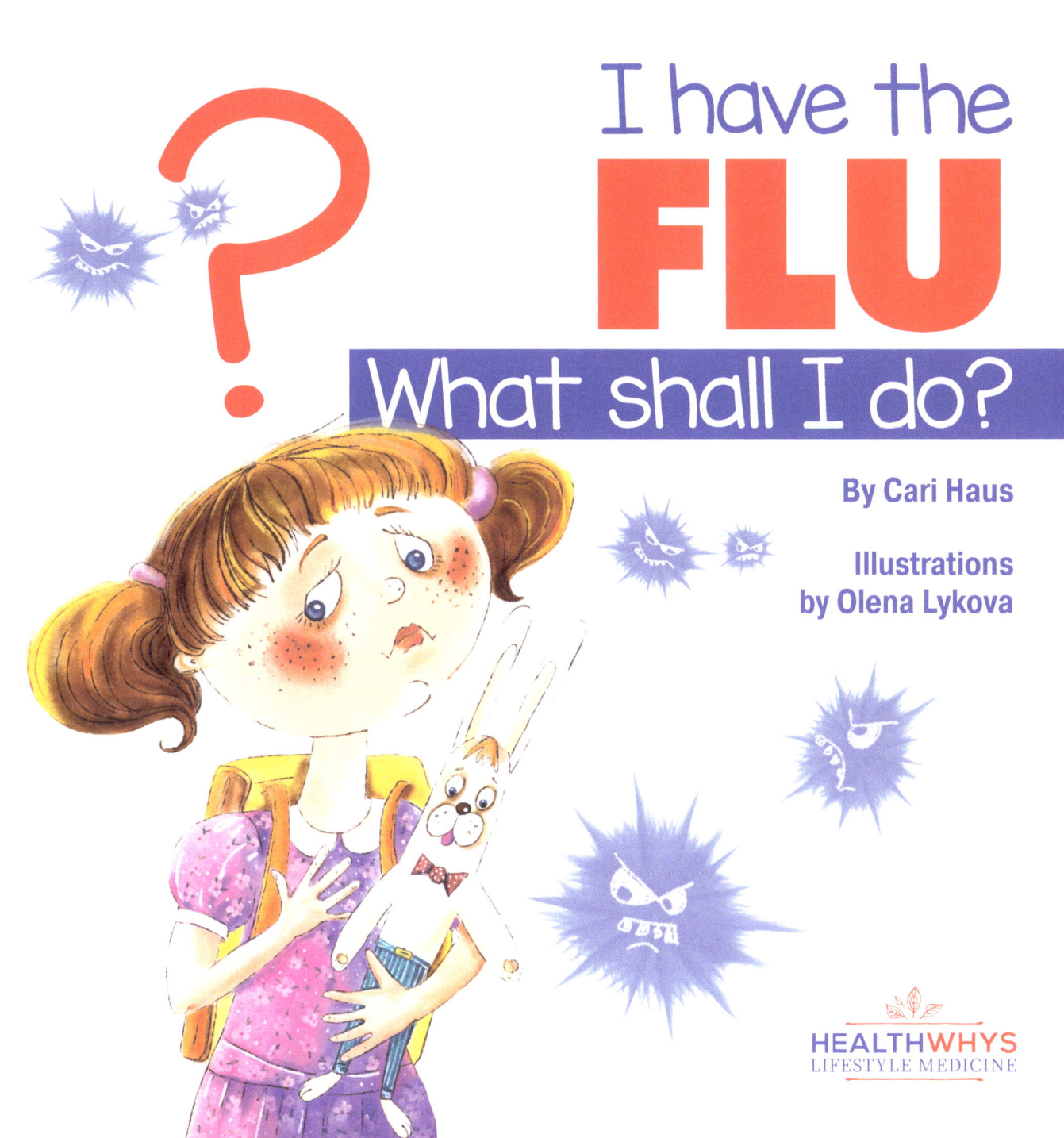

I have the FLU
What shall I do?

By Cari Haus

Illustrations by Olena Lykova

HEALTHWHYS
LIFESTYLE MEDICINE

Copyright © 2022 by:

HealthWhys Lifestyle Medicine
2363 Mountain Road
Hamburg, Pennsylvania 19526

All rights reserved. No part of this publication may be reproduced, distributed, or transmitted in any form or by any means, including photocopying, recording, or other electronic or mechanical methods, without the prior written permission of the publisher, except in the case of brief quotations embodied in critical reviews and certain other non-commercial uses permitted by copyright law. For permission or bulk copy requests, contact the publisher, addressed "Attention: Permissions Coordinator," at this address: info@healthwhys.com or call (610) 685-9900, or visit our website at http://www.healthwhys.com.

Author: Cari Haus
Illustrations and Interior Design: Olena Lykova

ISBN: 978-1-955866-00-2

This book contains the opinions and ideas of its authors. It is intended to provide helpful general information on he subjects that it addresses. It is not in any way a substitute for the advice of the reader's own physician(s) or other medical professionals based on the reader's own individual conditions, symptoms, or concerns. If the reader needs personal medical, health, dietary, exercise, or other assistance or advice, the reader should consult a competent physician and/or other qualified health care professionals. The author and publisher specifically disclaim all responsibility for injury, damage, or loss that the reader may incur as a direct or indirect consequence of following any direction or suggestions given in this book or participating in any programs described in this book.

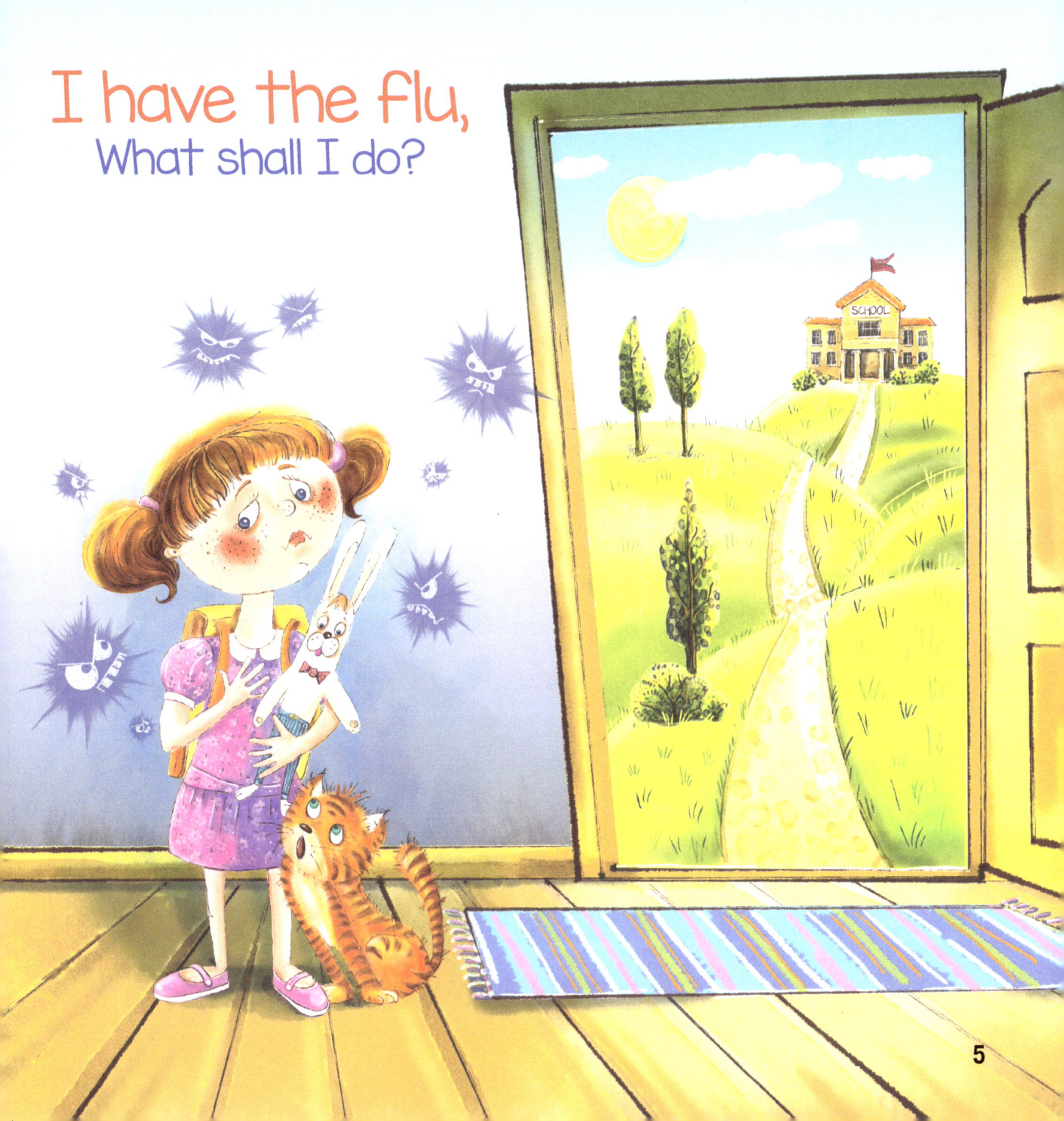

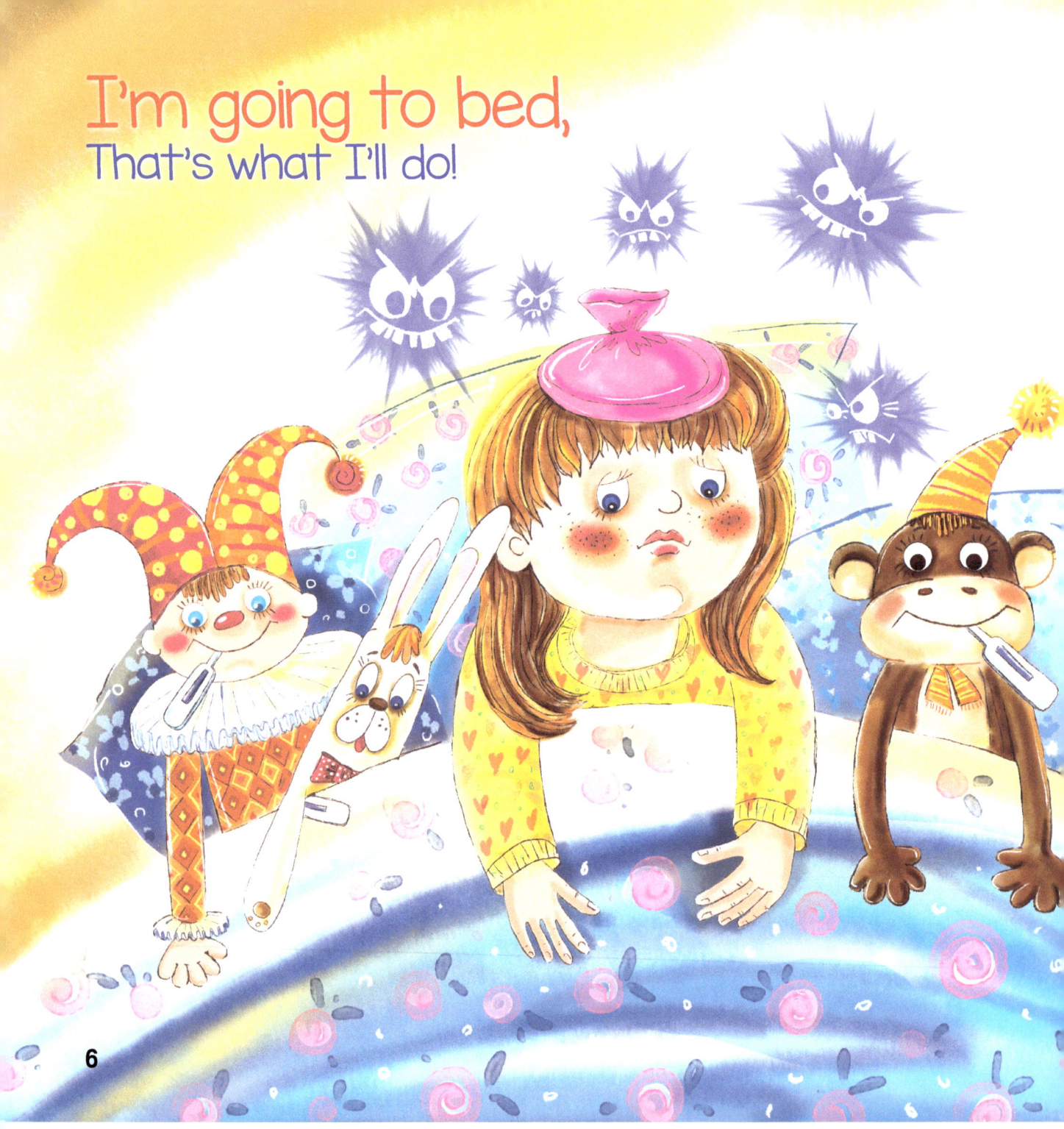

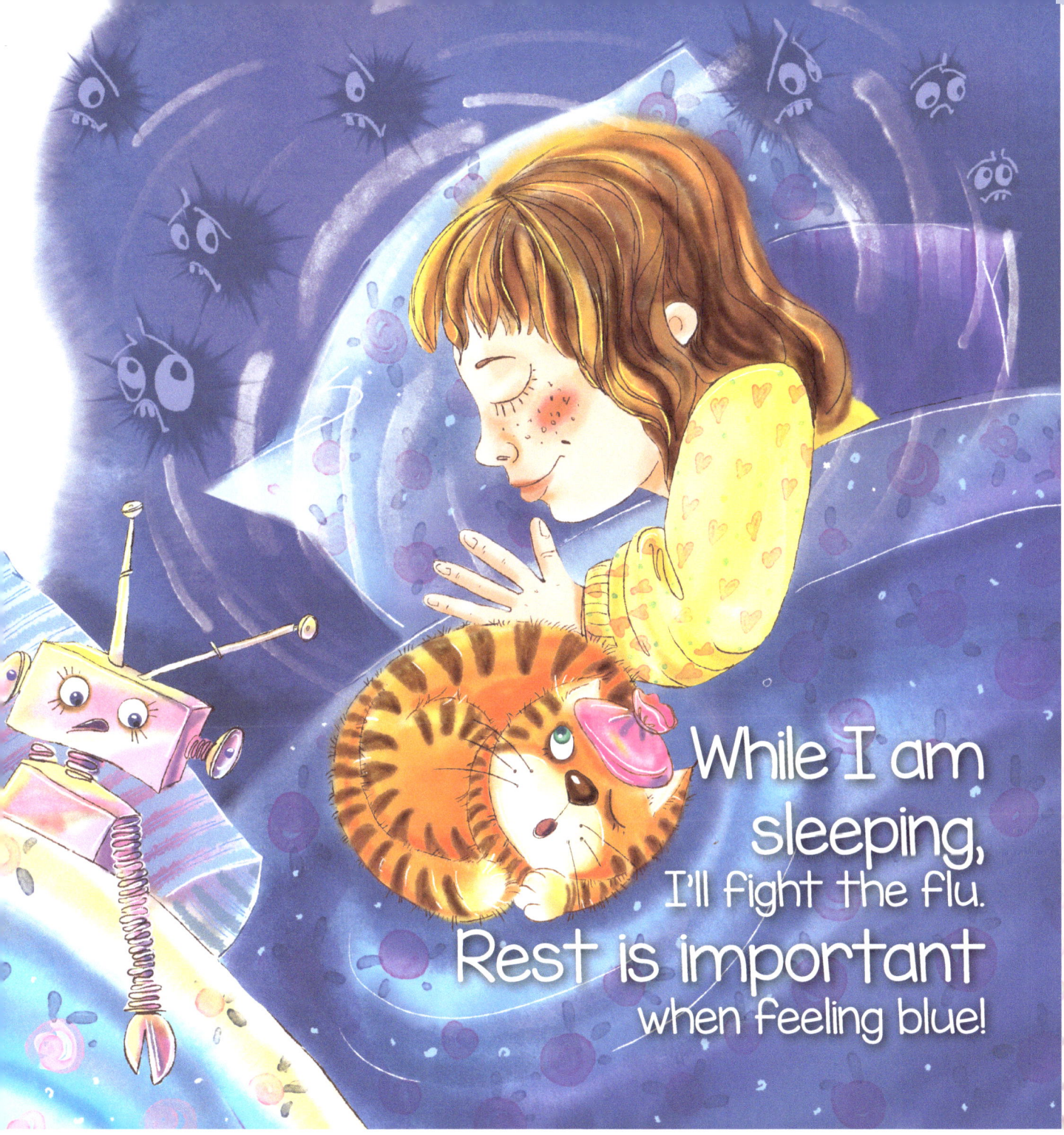

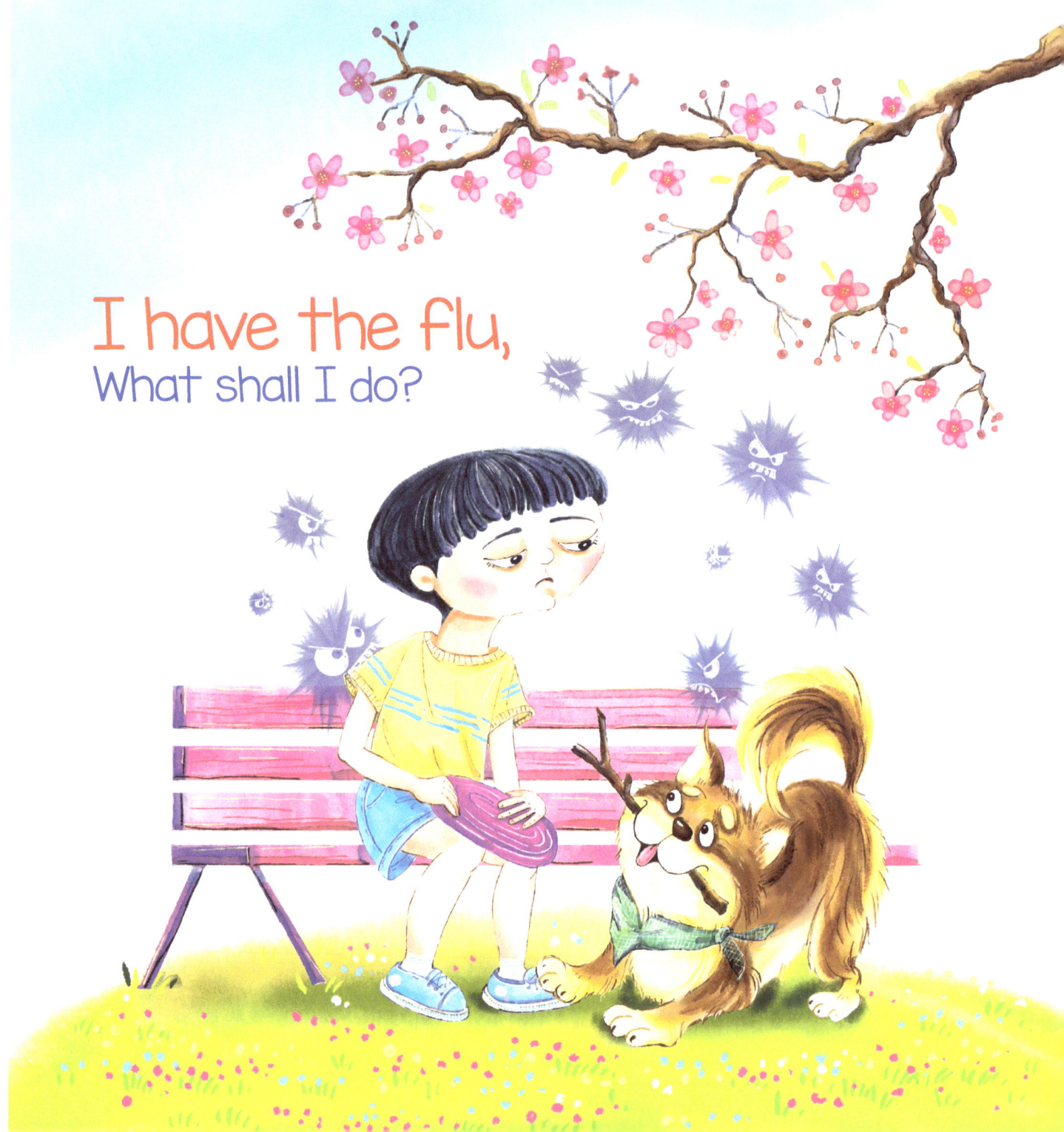

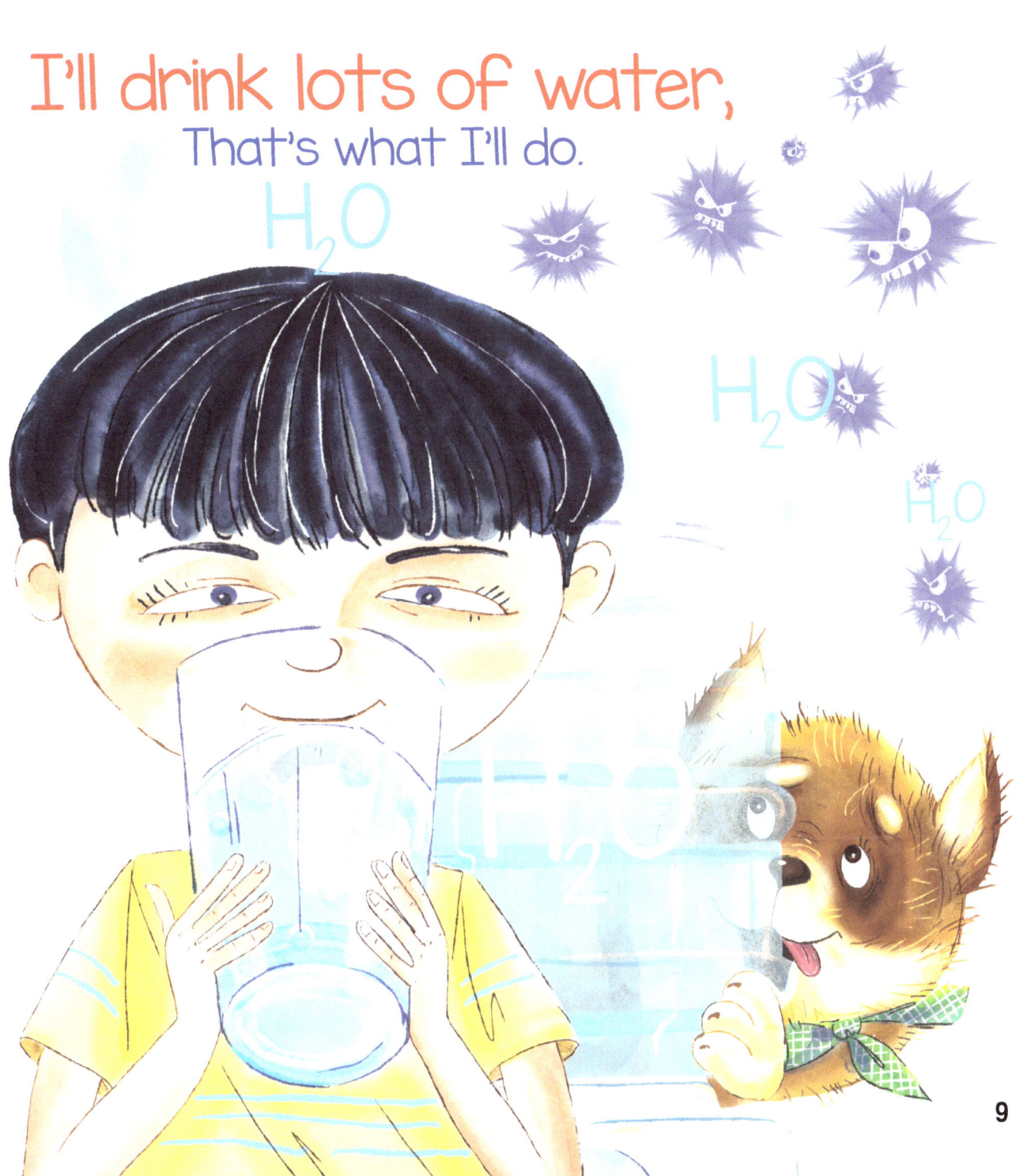

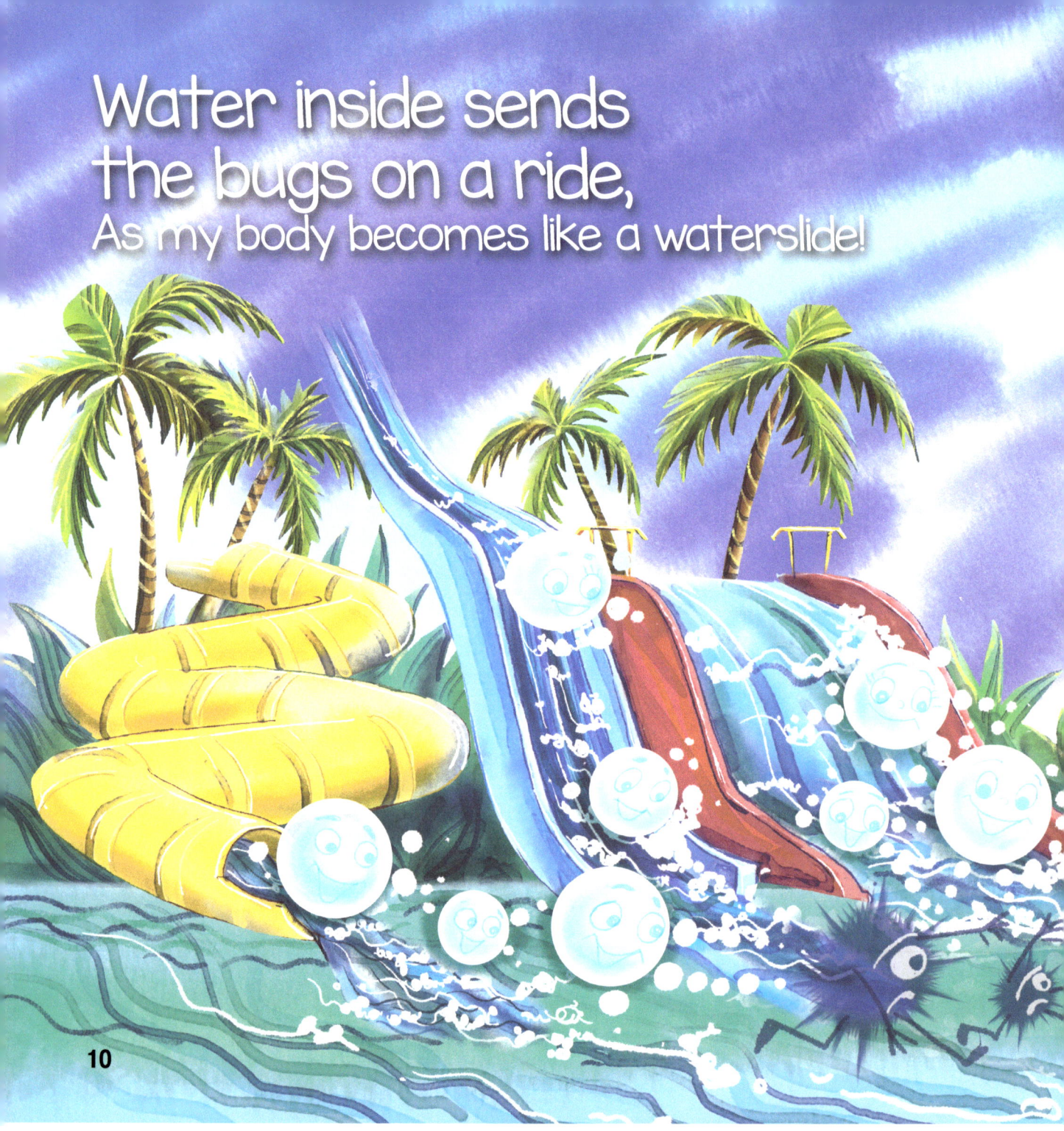
Water inside sends the bugs on a ride,
As my body becomes like a waterslide!

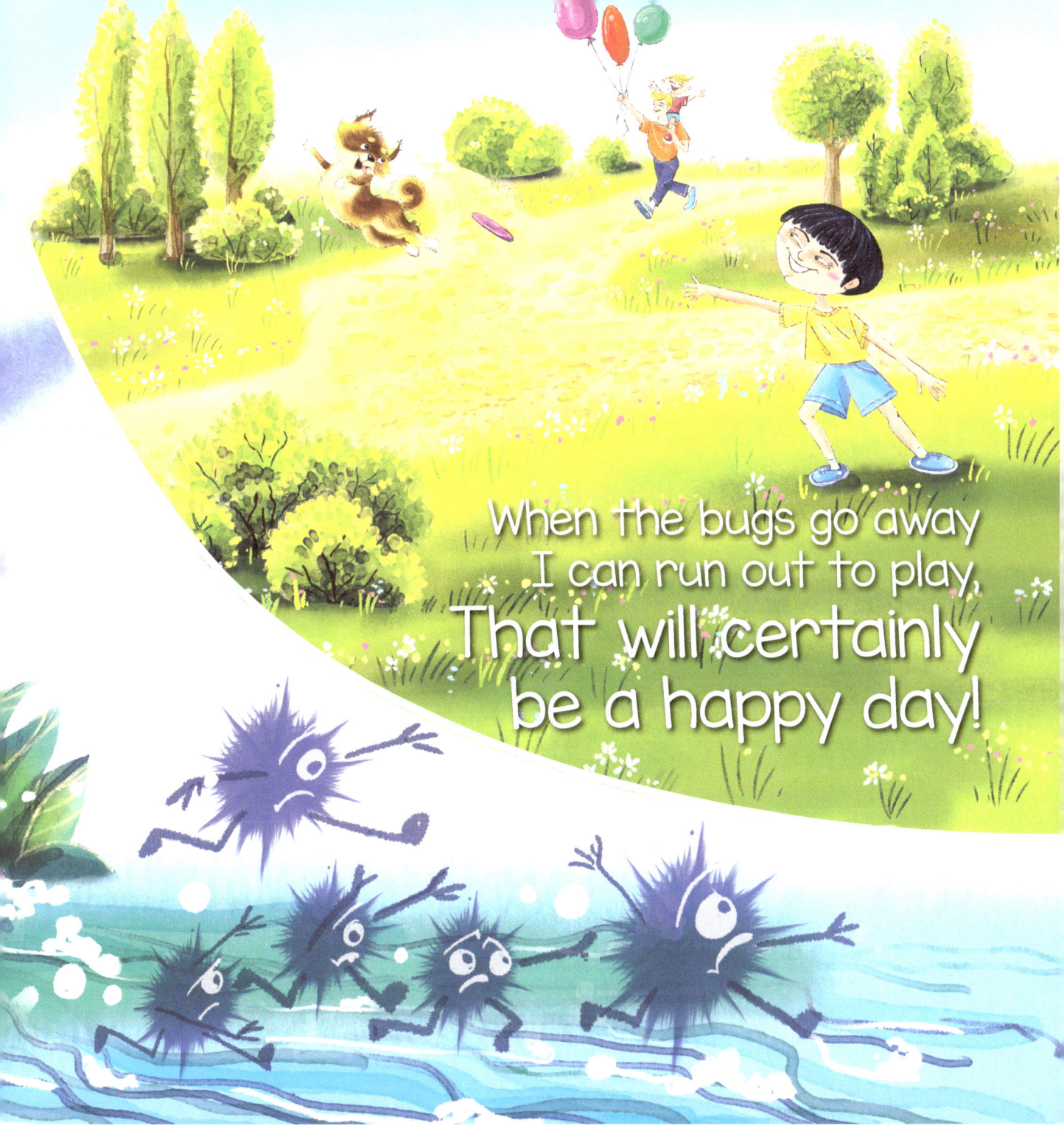
When the bugs go away
I can run out to play,
That will certainly
be a happy day!

Water on my outside can be helpful too.

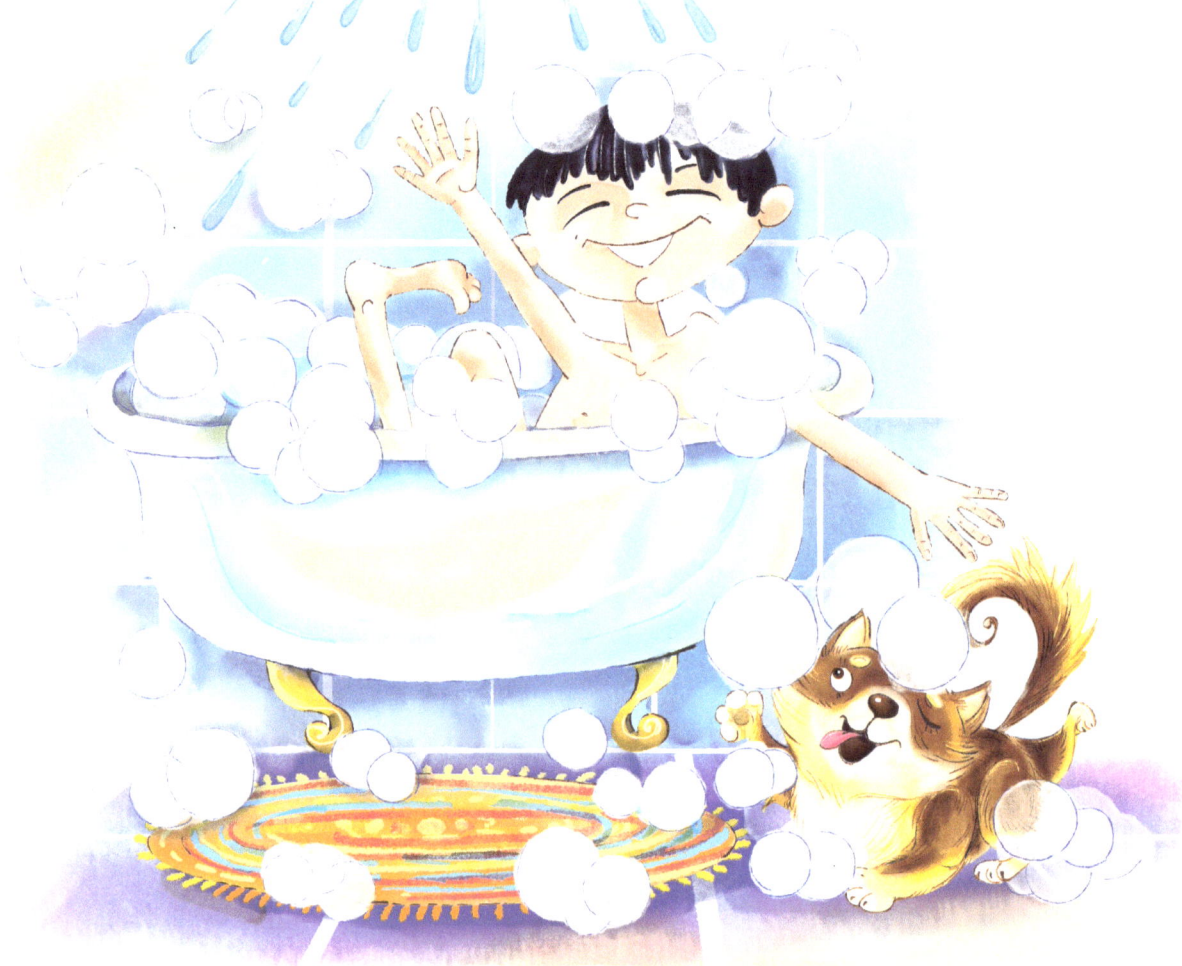

A sauna or shower or dipsy-do
In a nice warm tub can help fight the flu!

I have the flu, what shall I eat?
Should I have fries or something sweet?

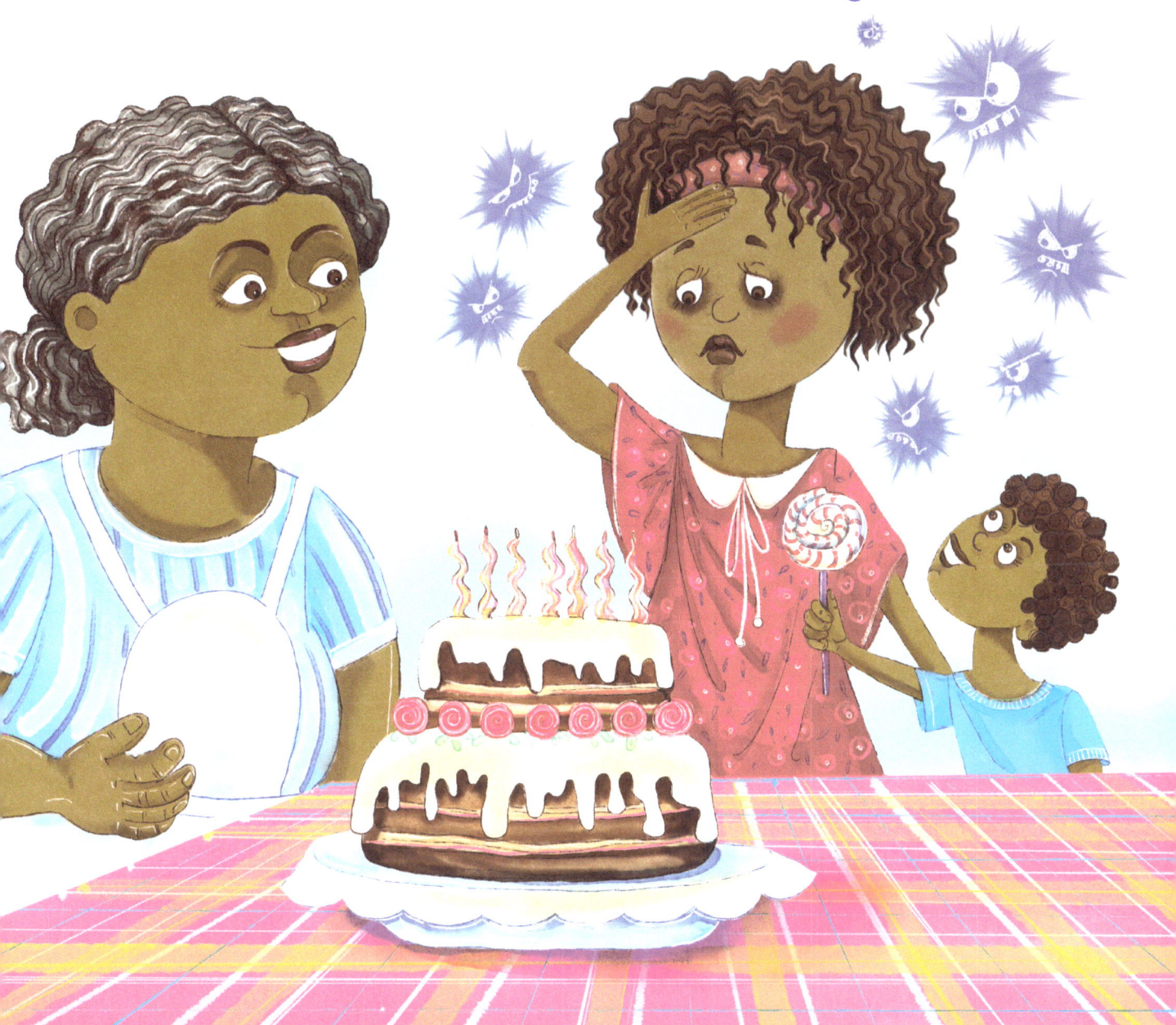

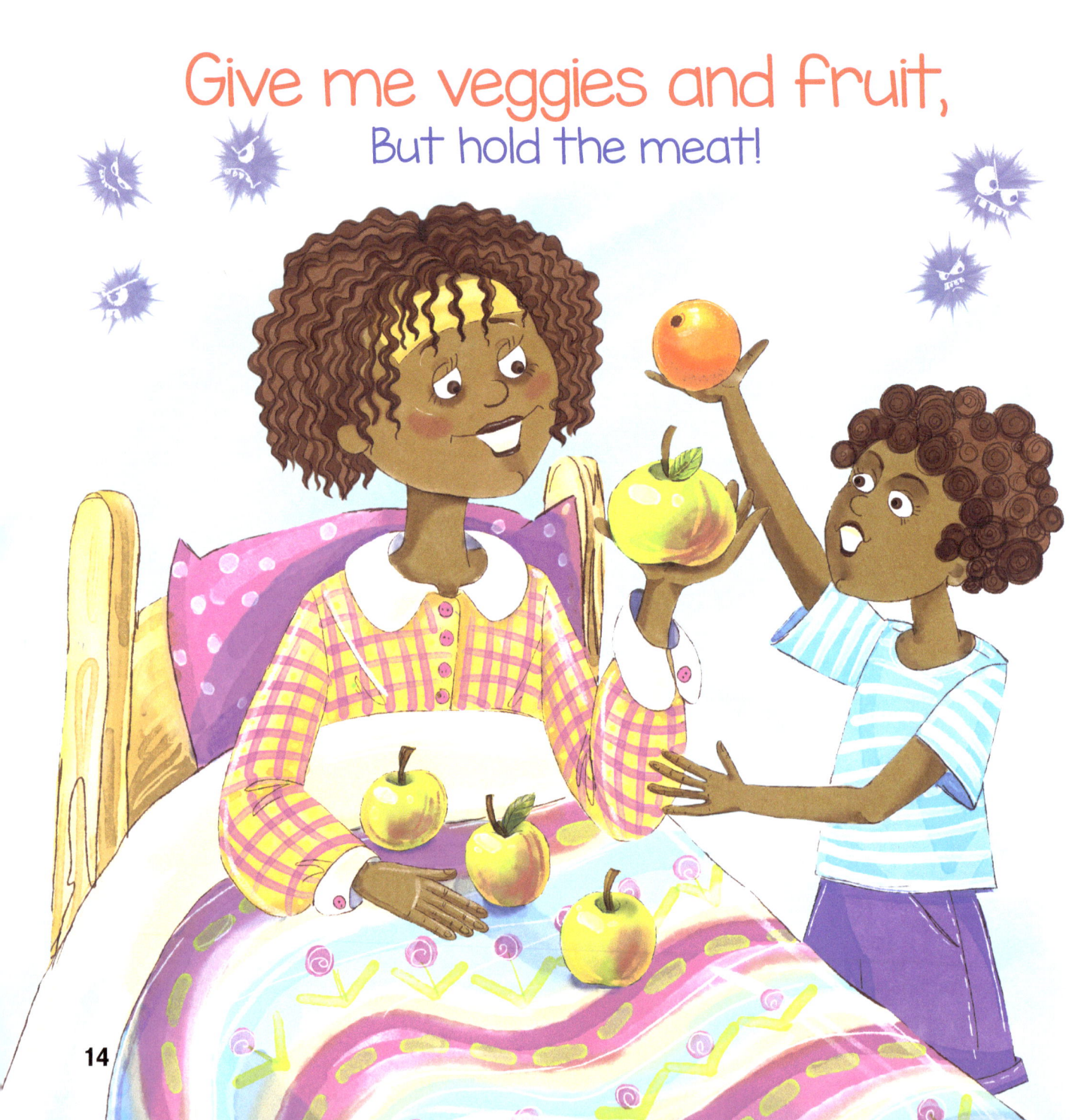

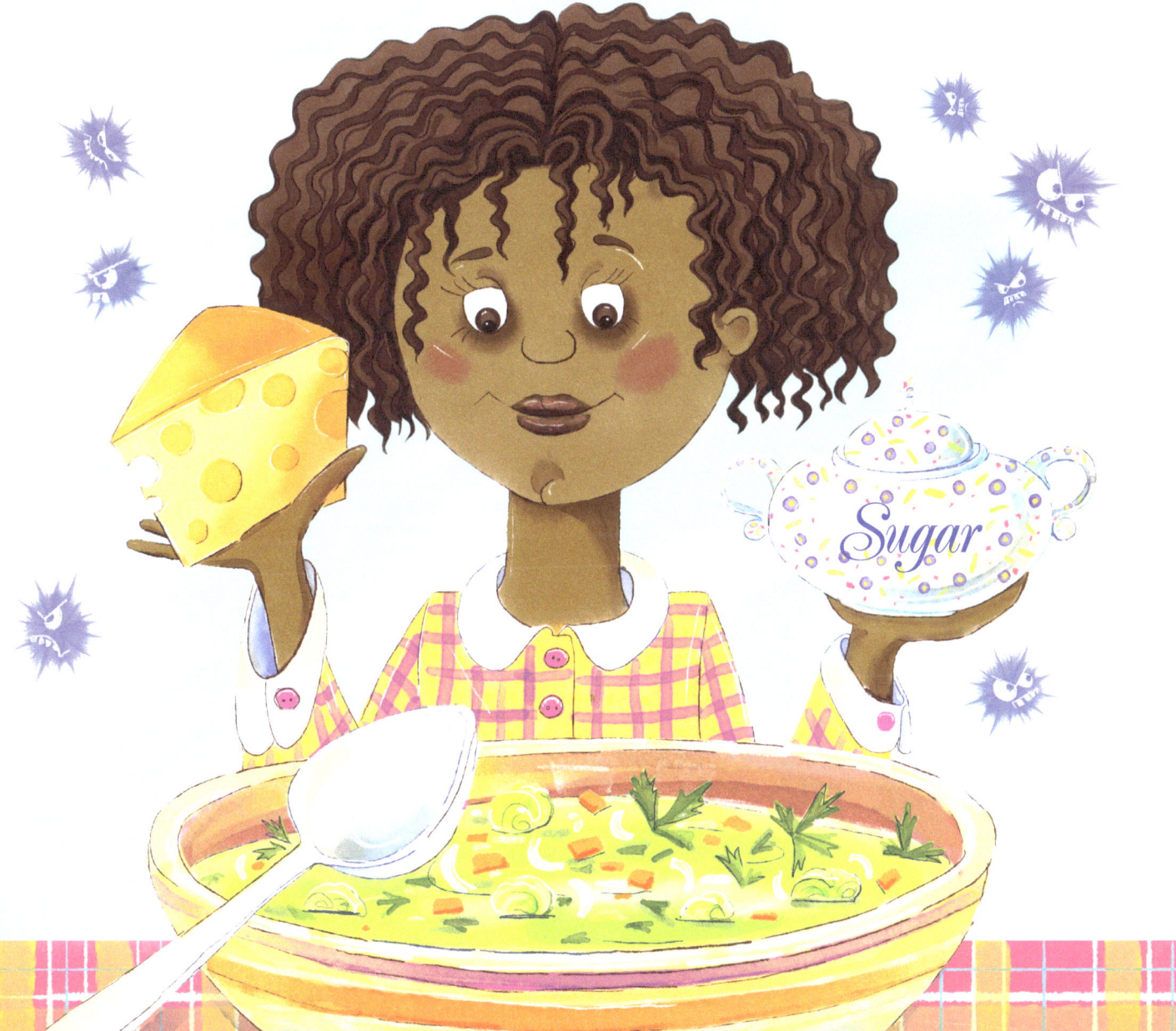

If food is greasy or hard to digest,
I won't eat it now—
That just wouldn't be best!

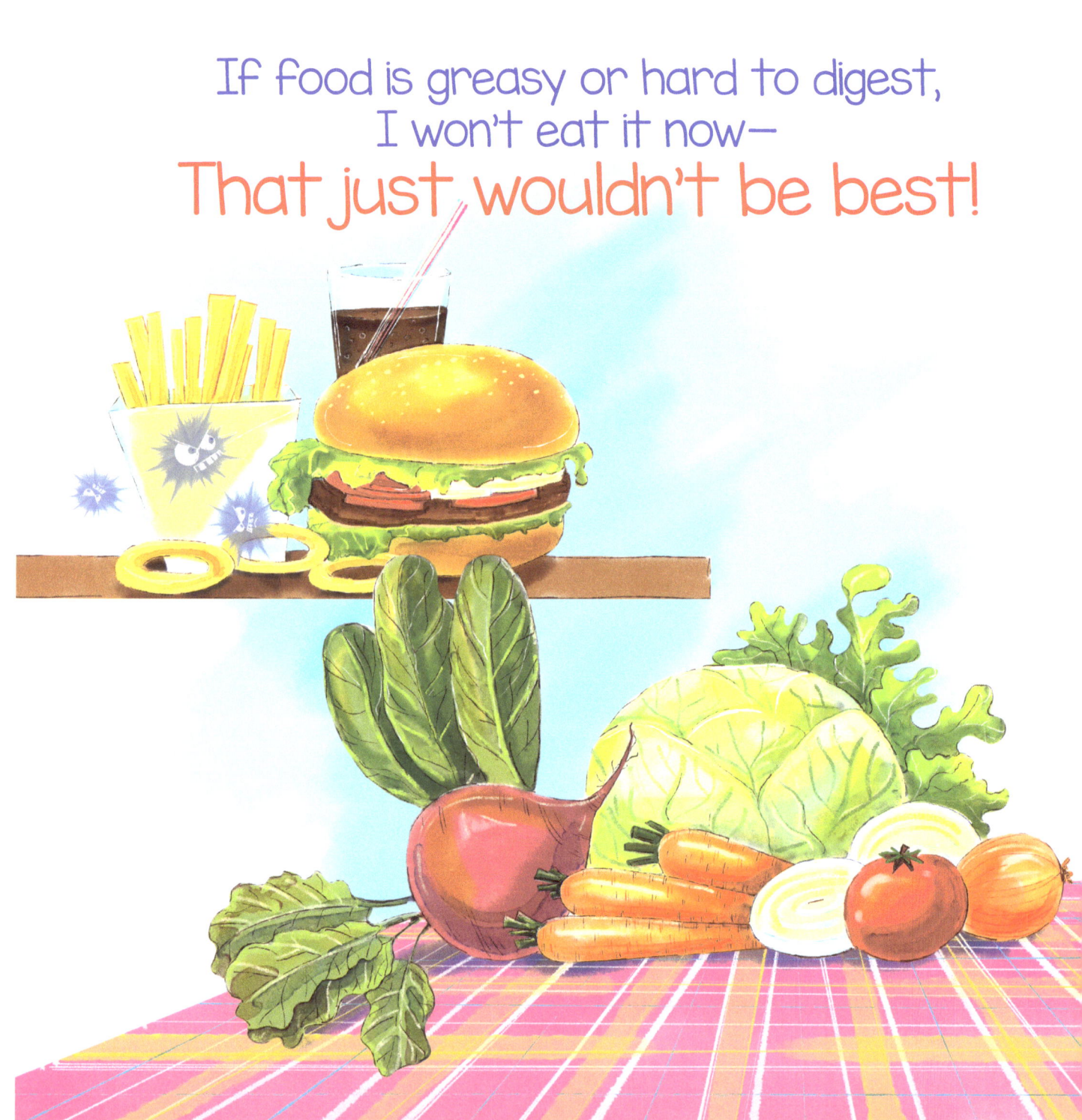

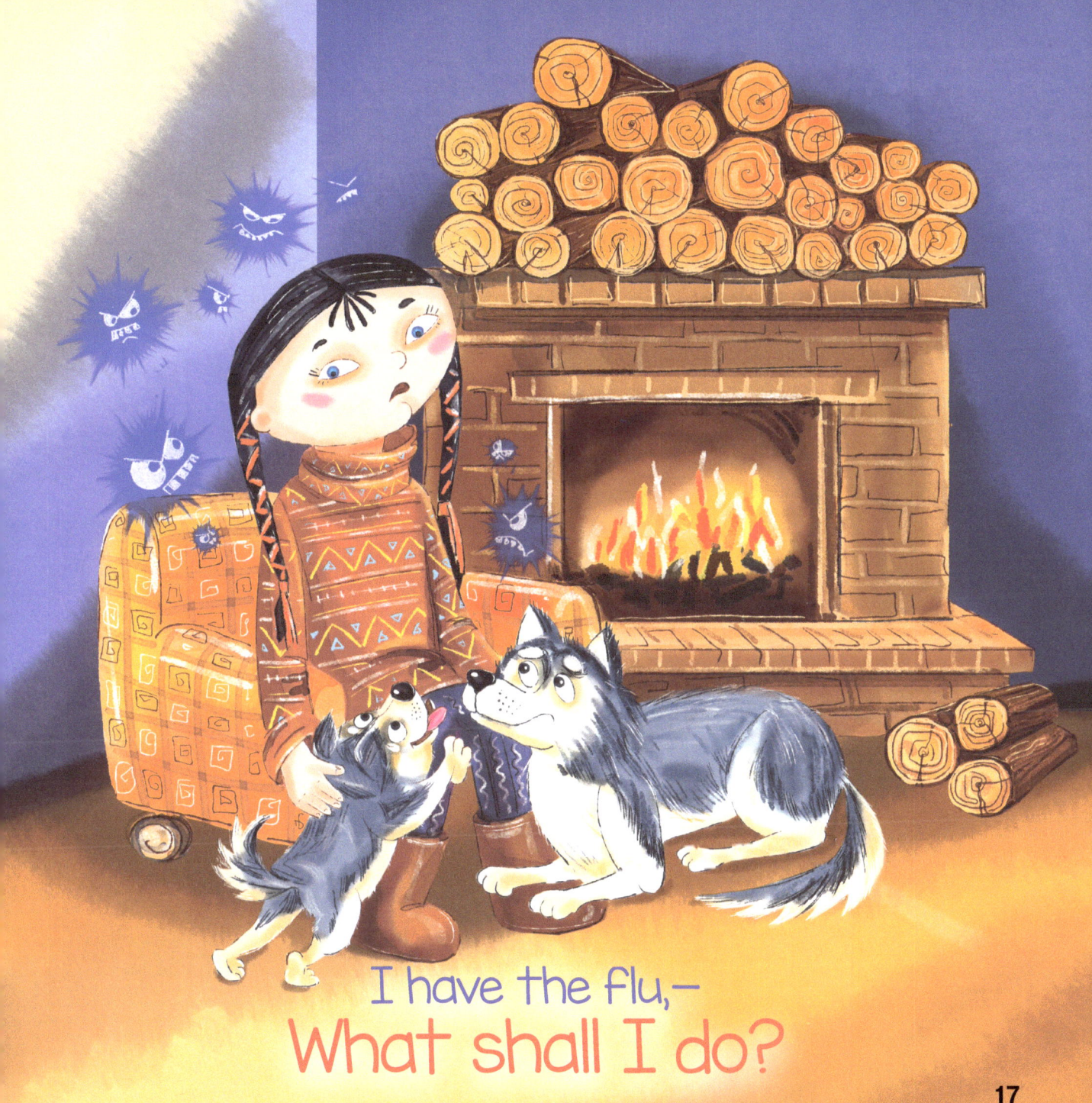

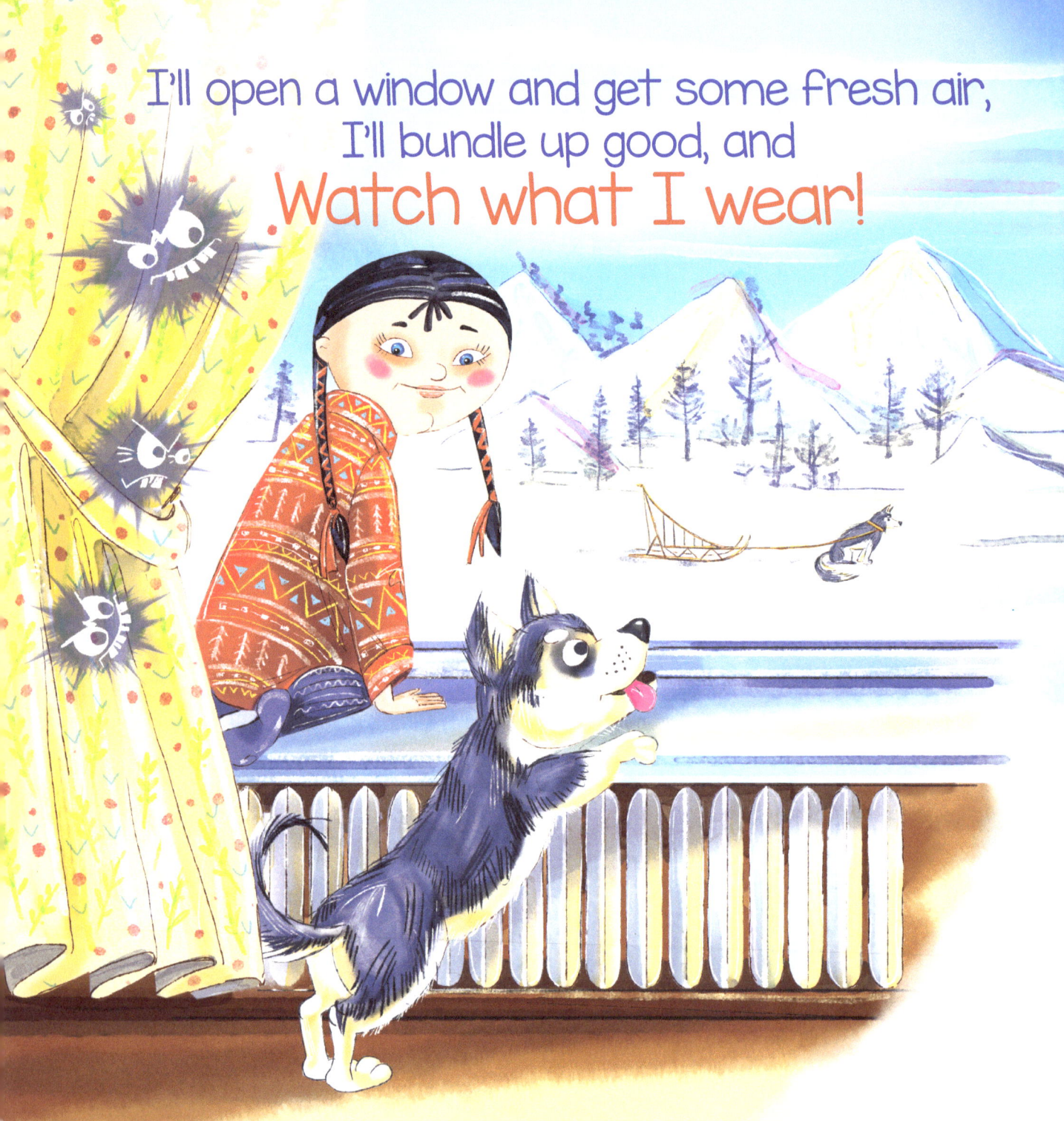

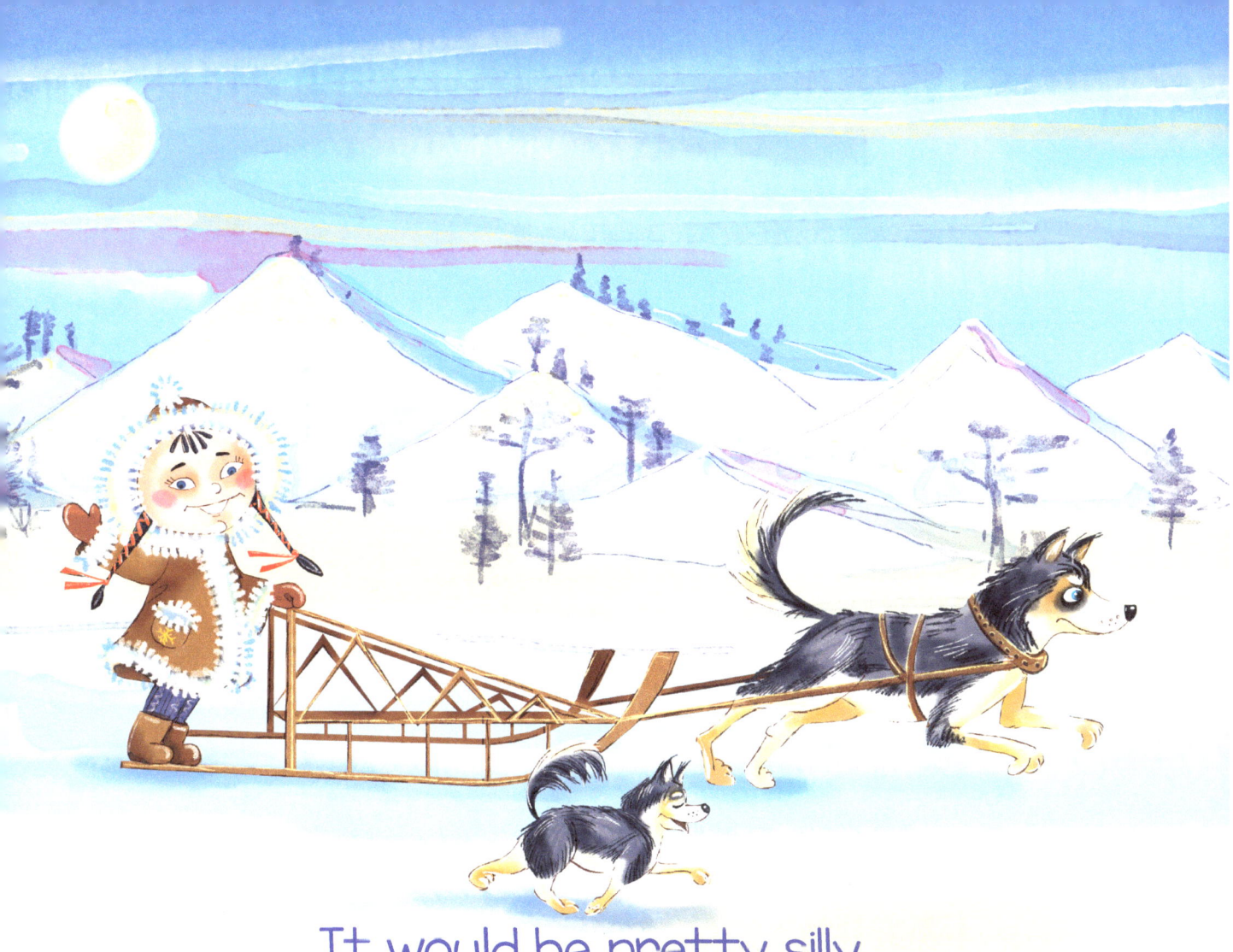

It would be pretty silly
To get myself chilly,
When I'm fighting the flu,
That's a bad thing to do!

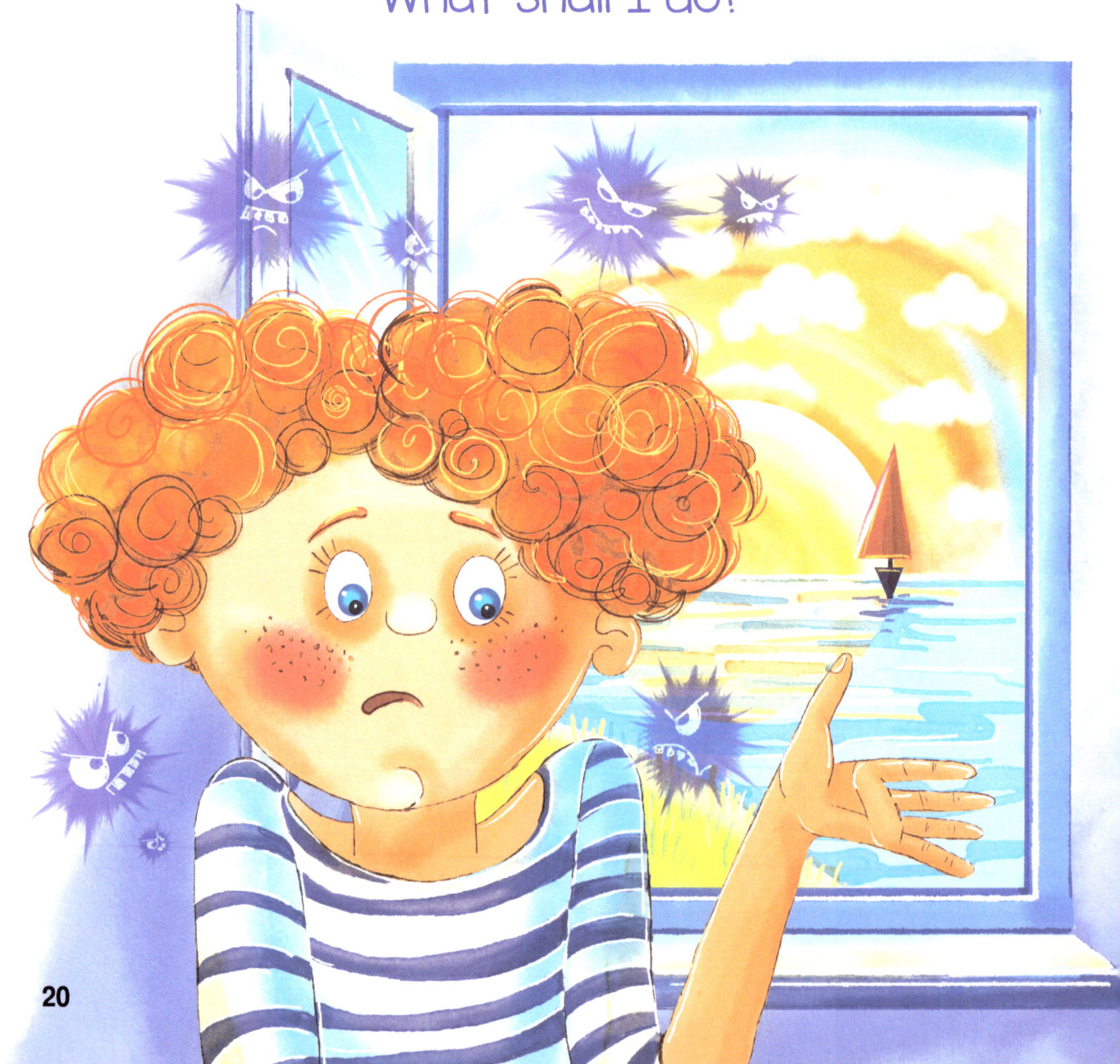

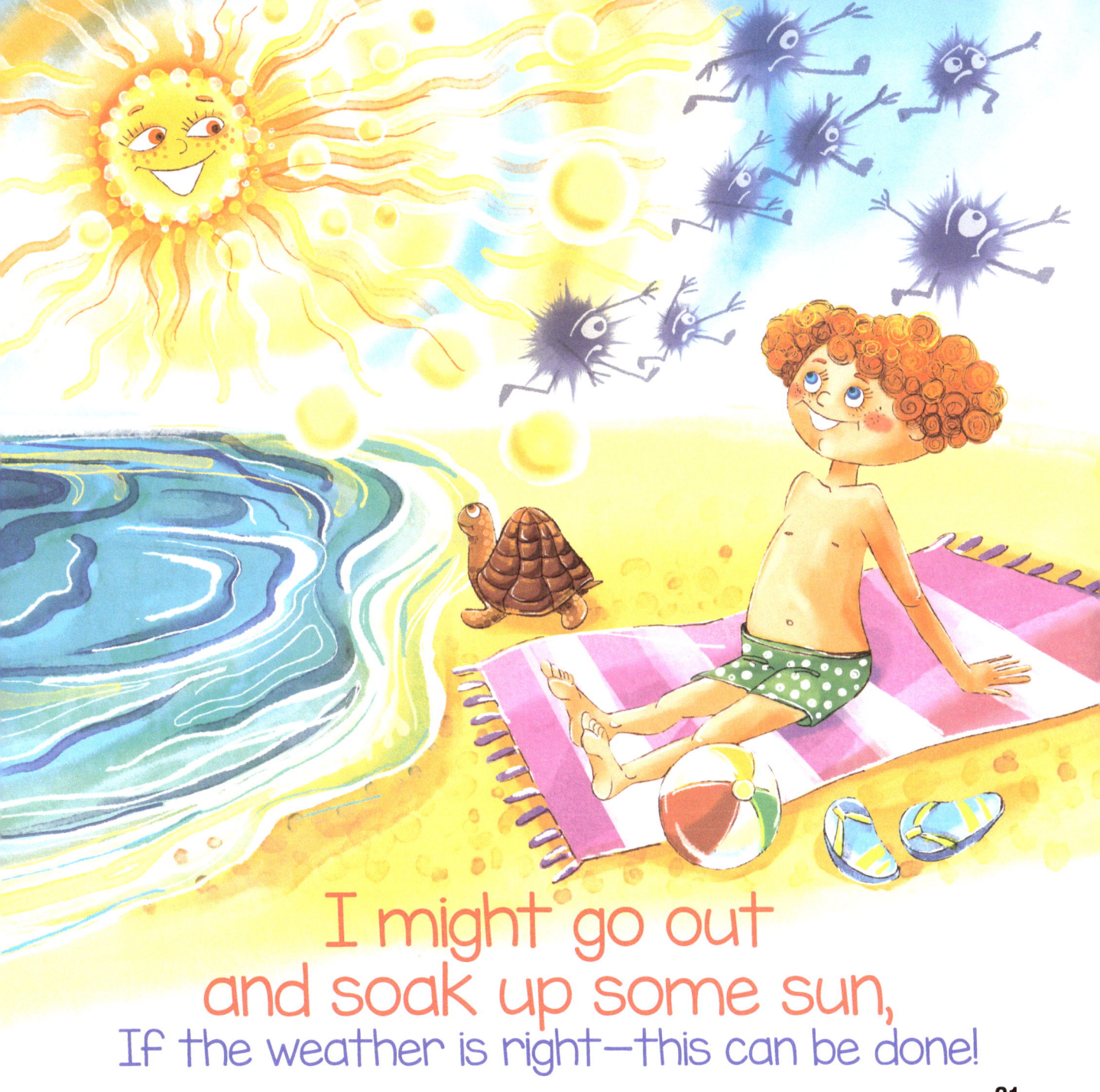

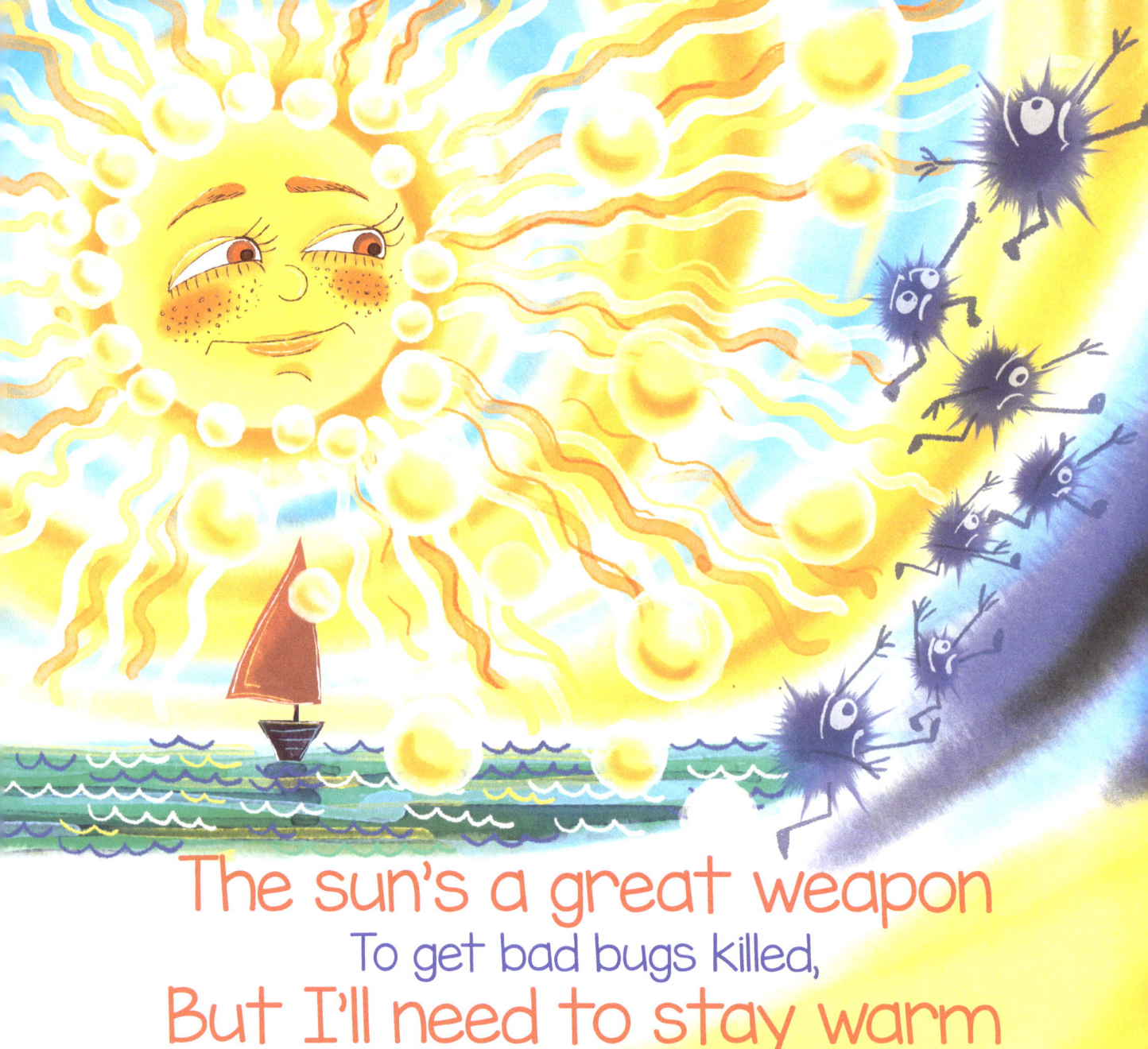

The sun's a great weapon
To get bad bugs killed,
But I'll need to stay warm
And not get chilled!

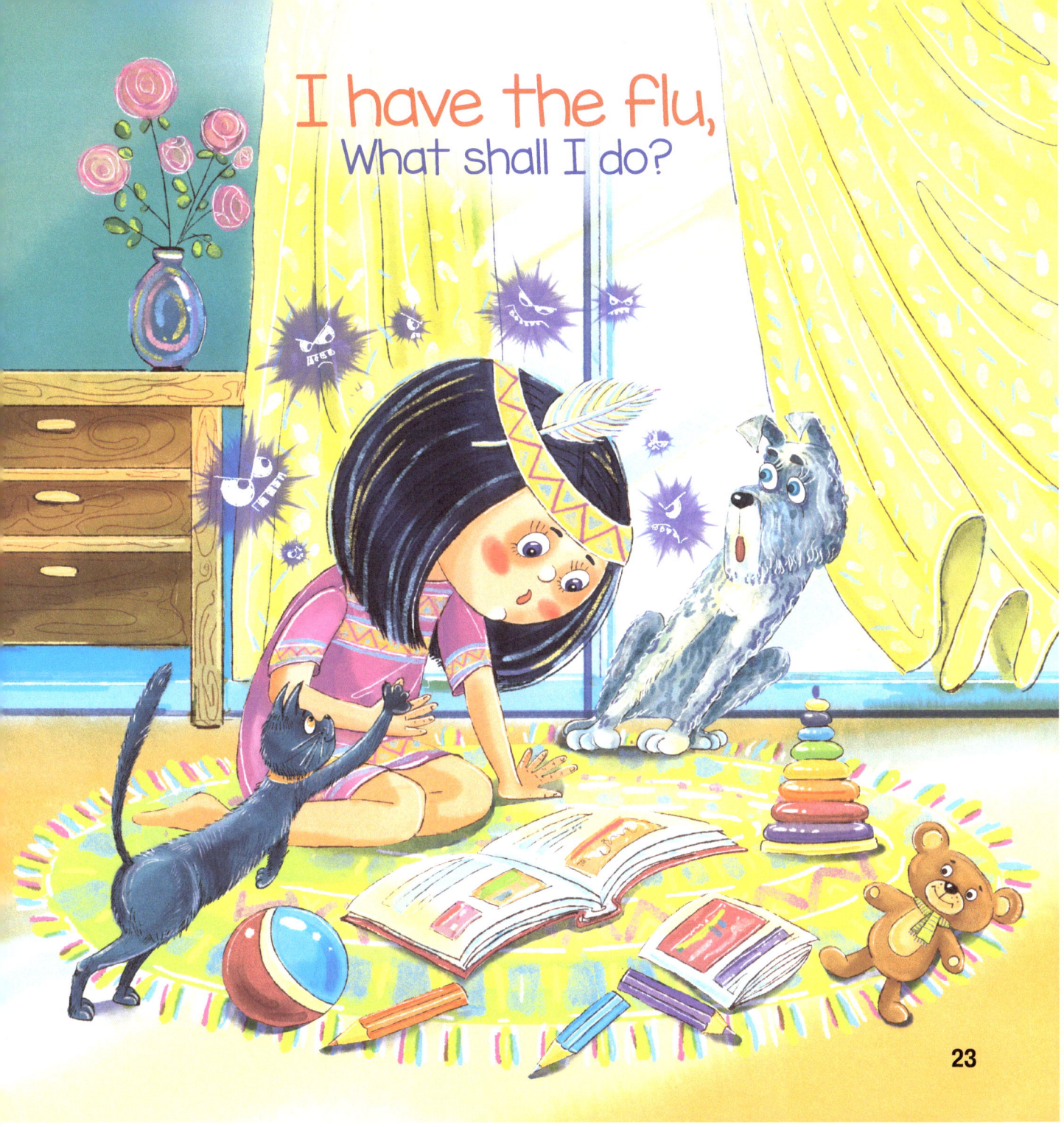

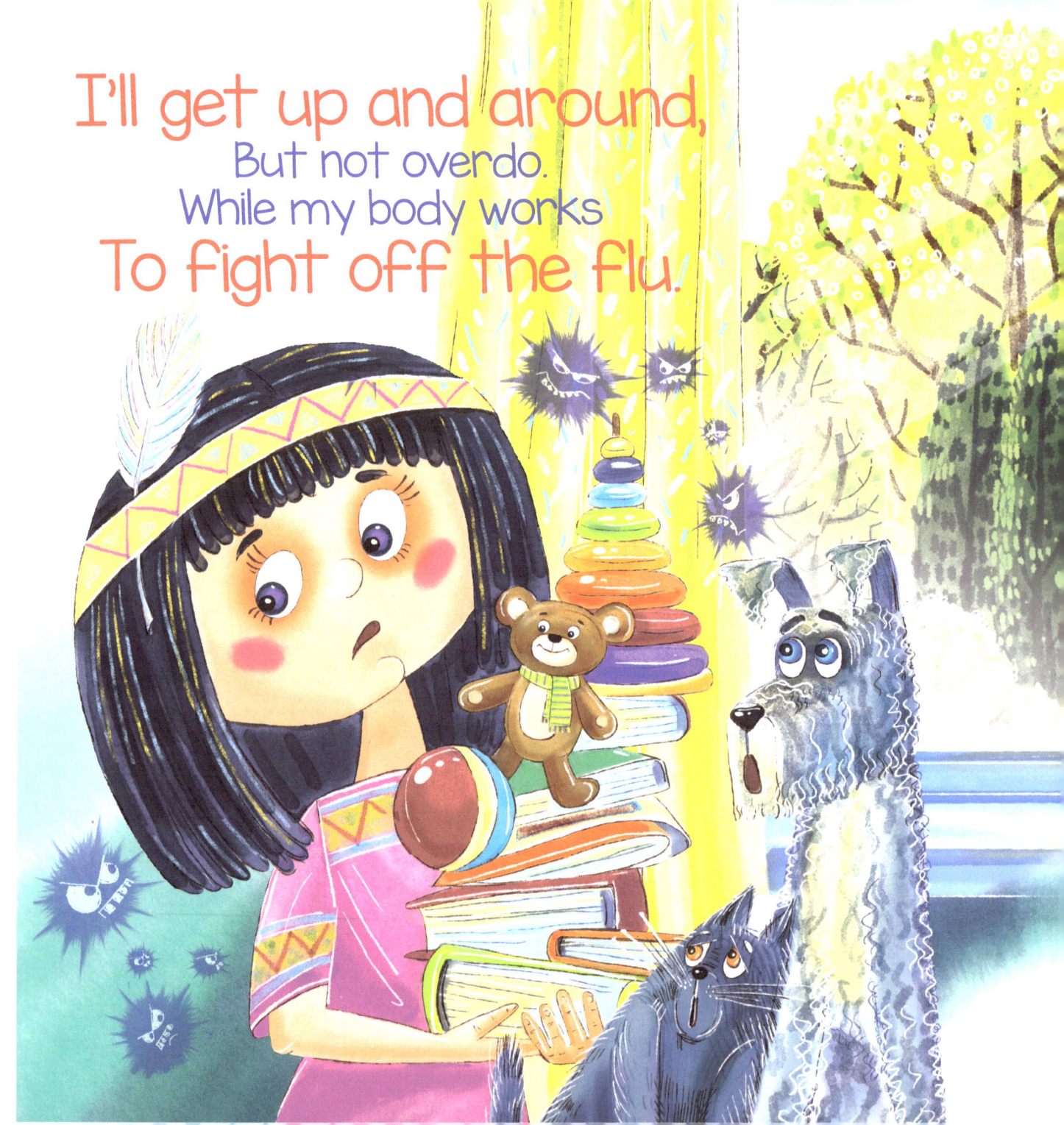

I'll get up and around,
But not overdo.
While my body works
To fight off the flu.

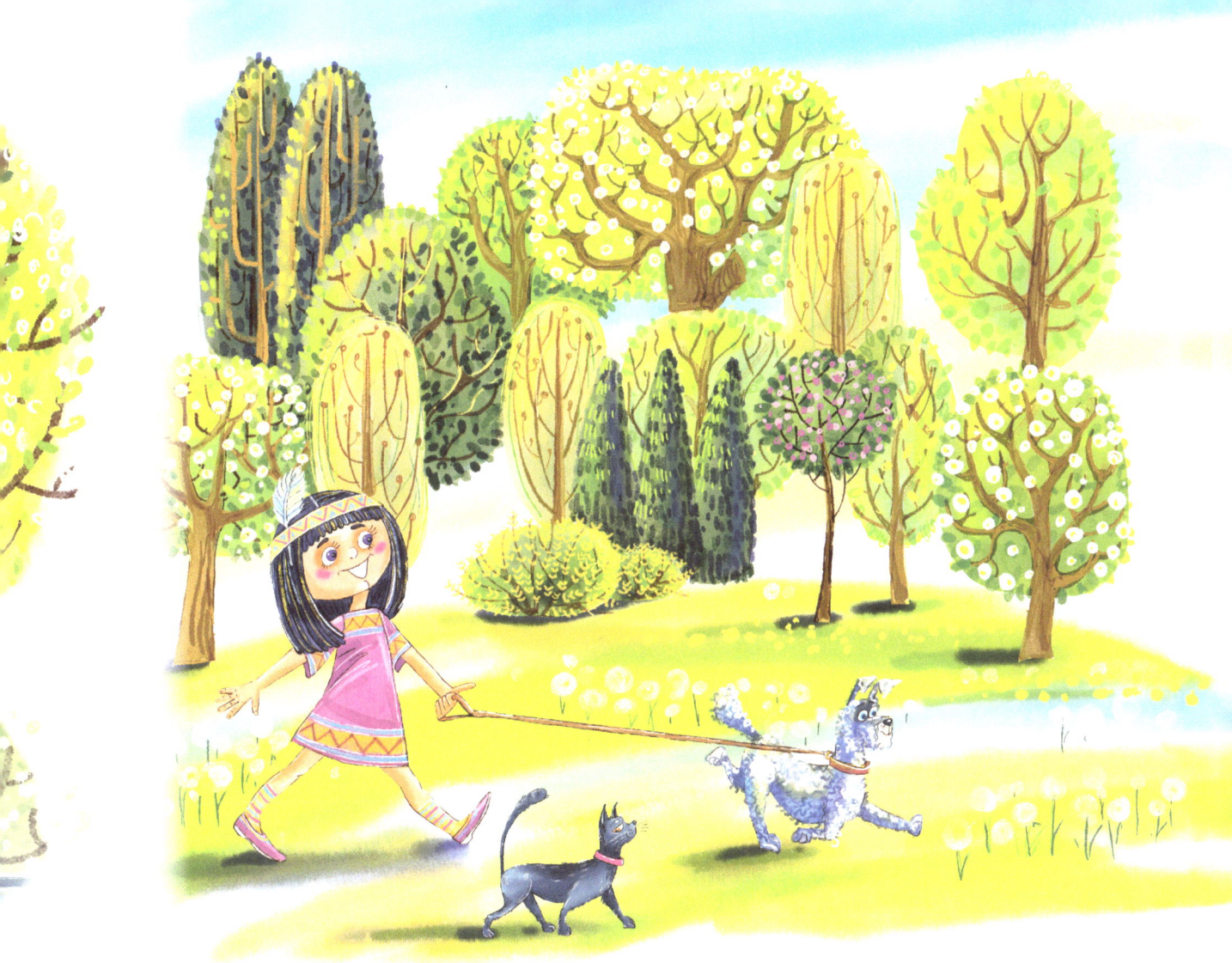

It's not good to be a total couch 'tater,
But running a mile
Should be saved for later!

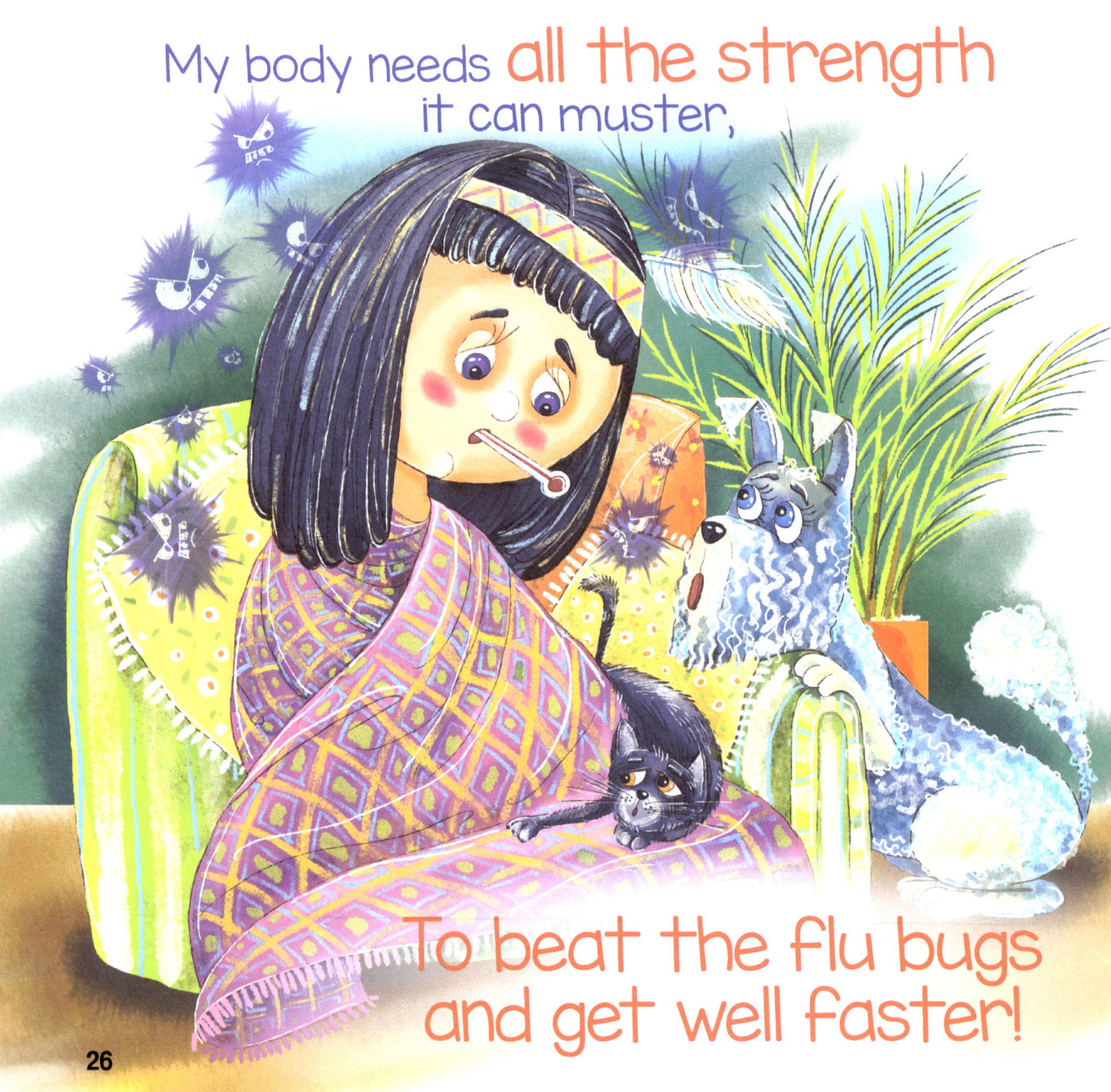

If I keep getting worse,
We won't wait for a scare,
It's time to go get some medical care!

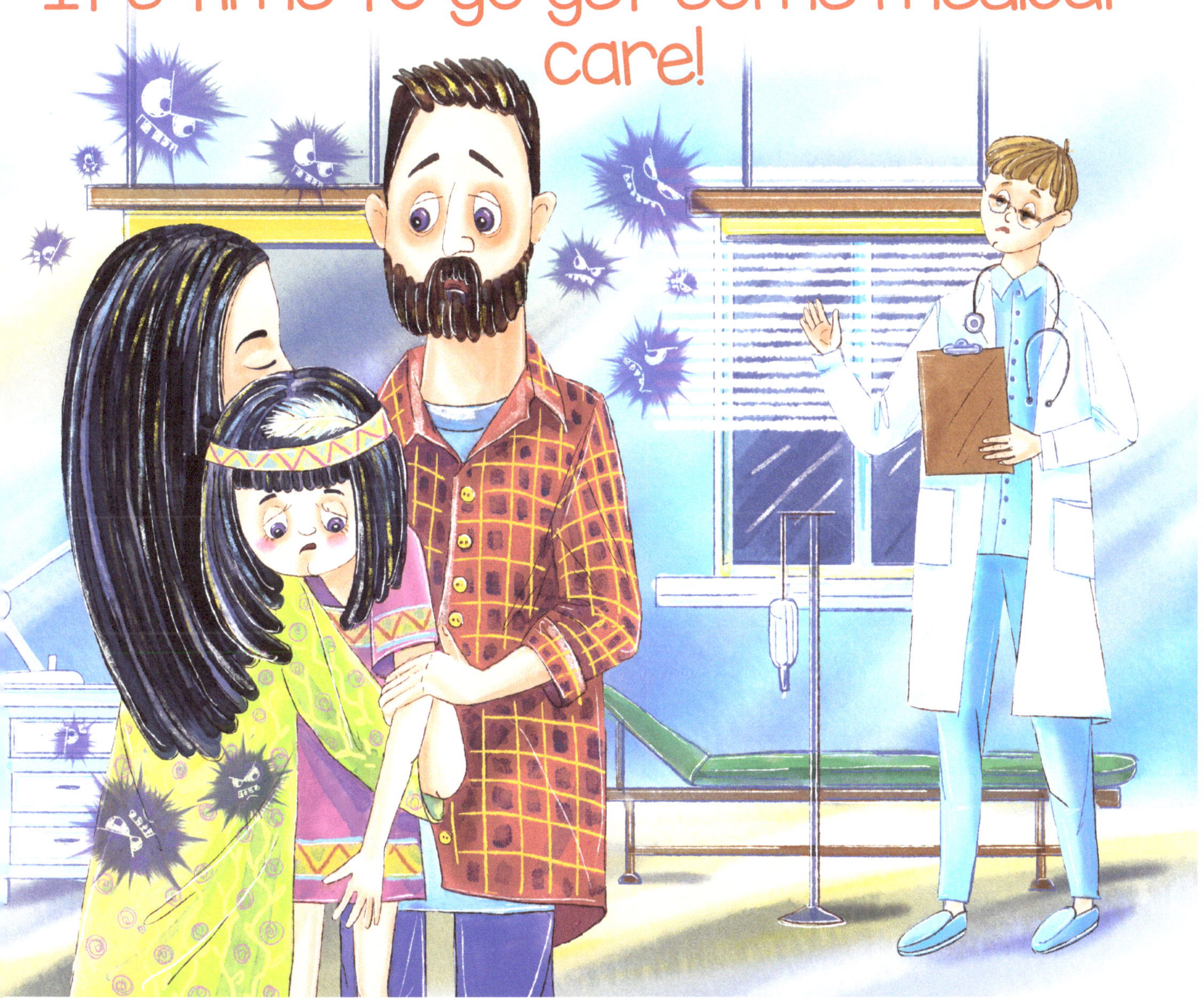

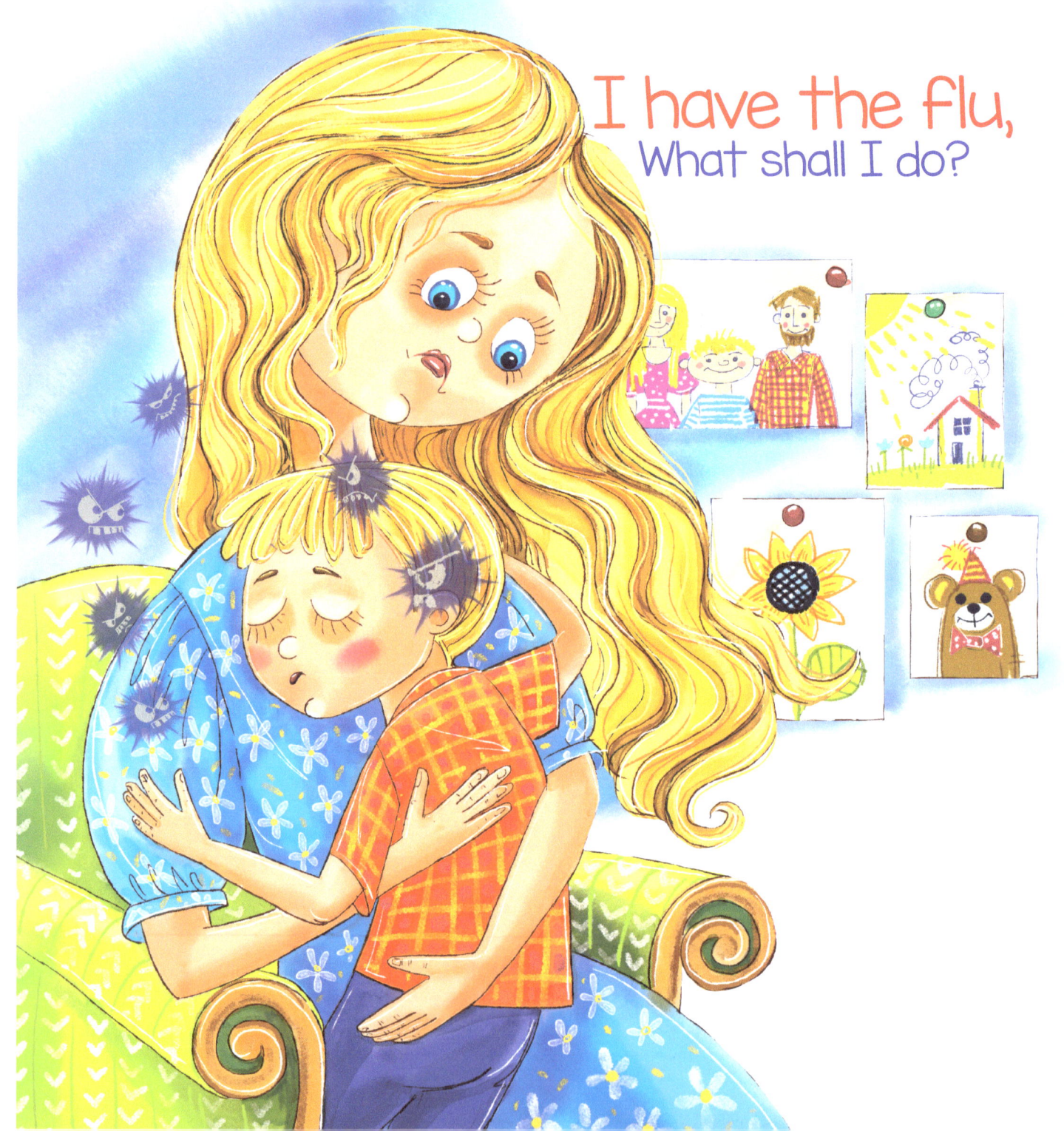

I'll try to be happy-remember to smile, and think,
"I will be better in a little while."

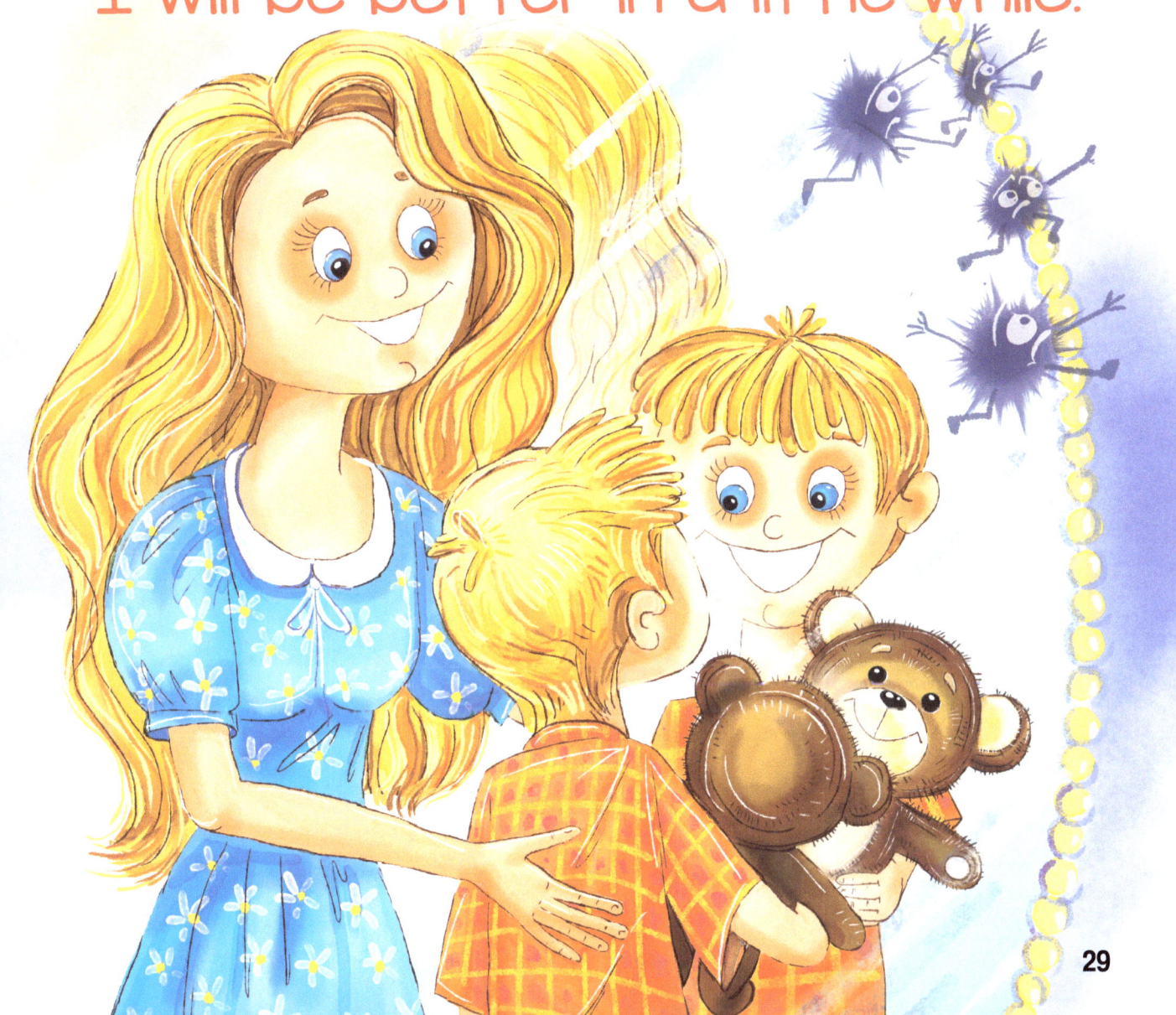

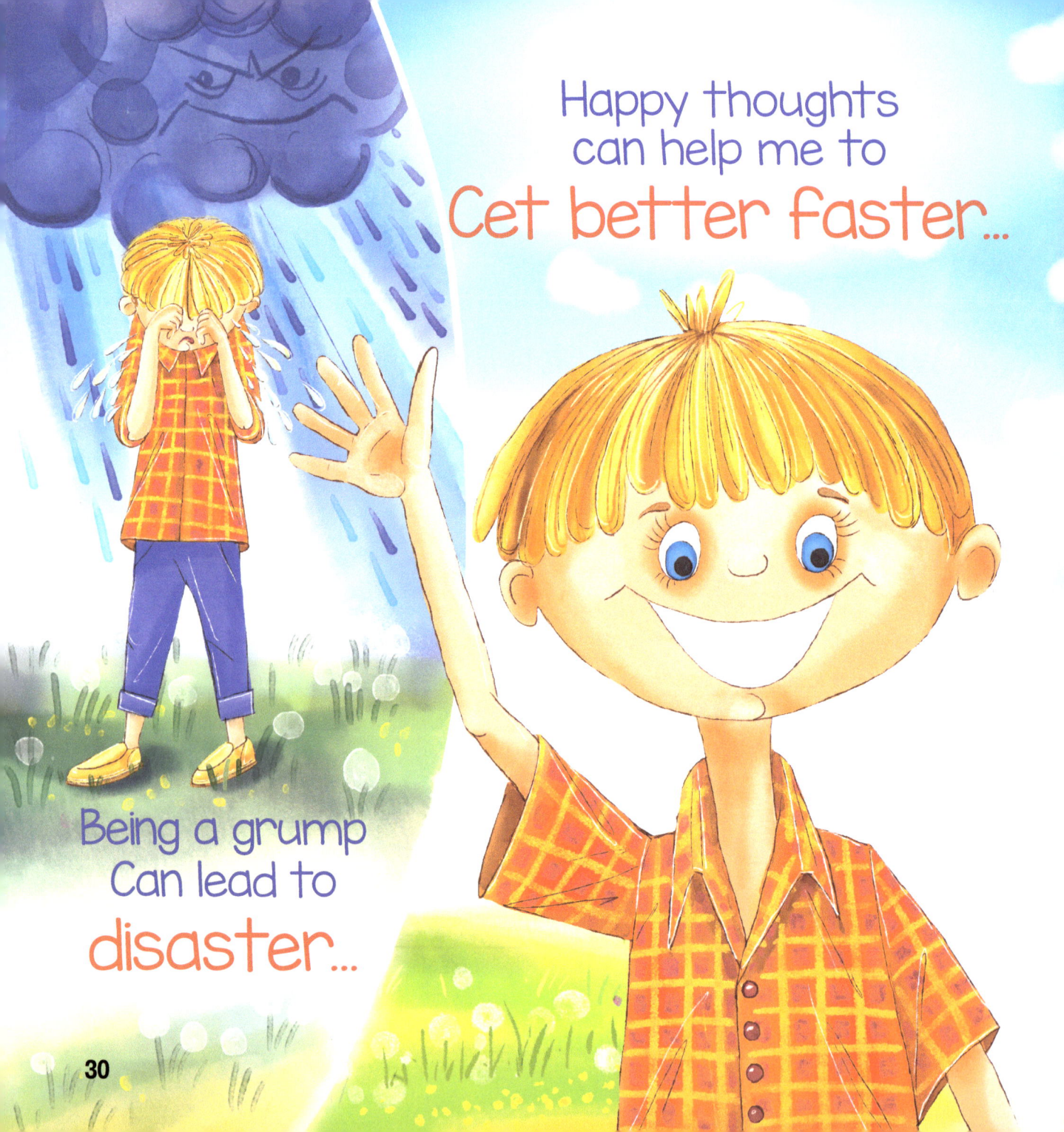

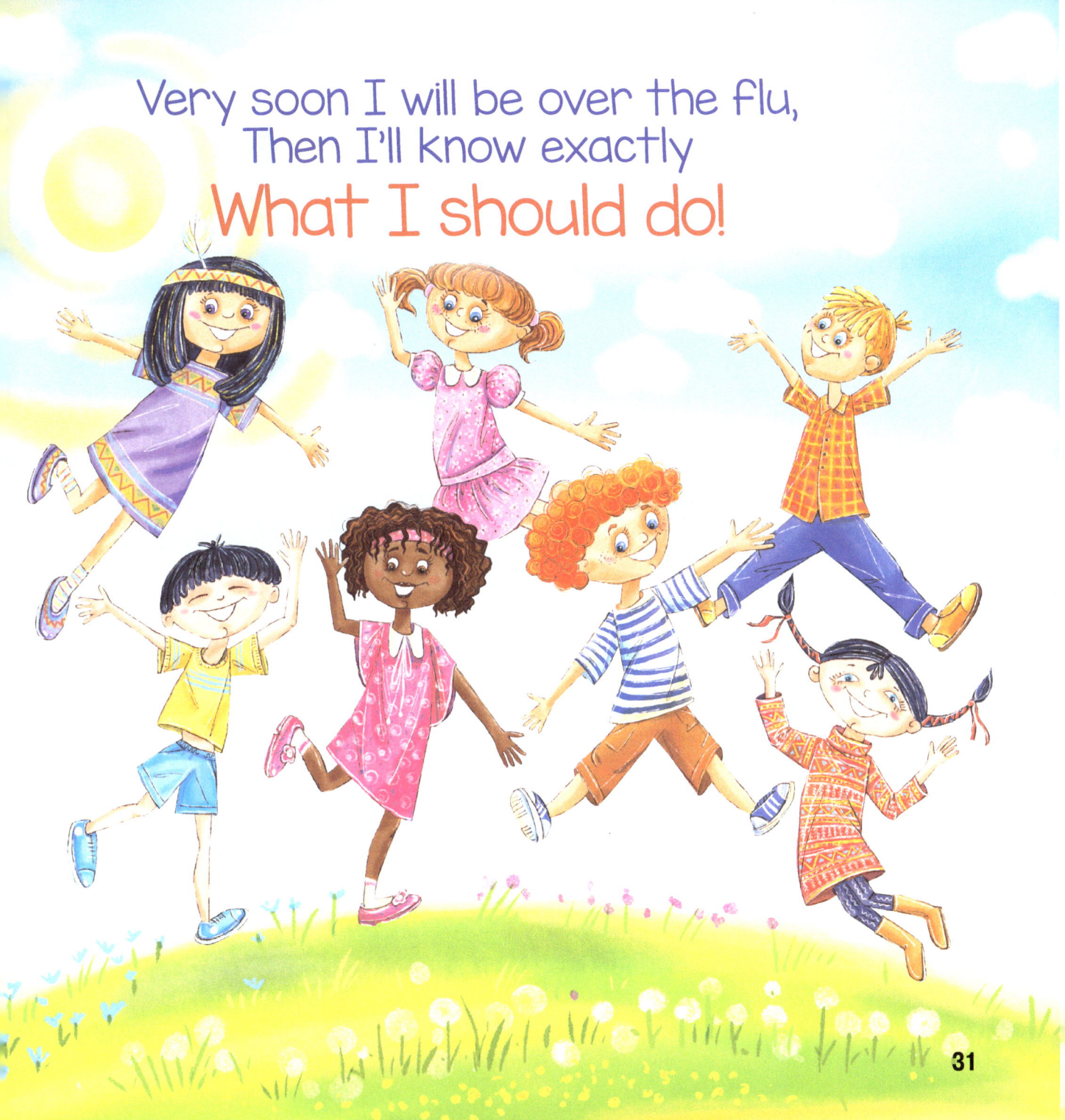

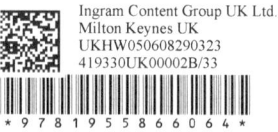
Ingram Content Group UK Ltd.
Milton Keynes UK
UKHW050608290323
419330UK00002B/33